CONTENTS

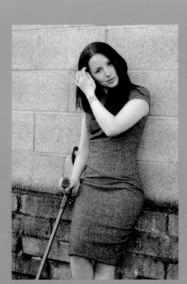

Text by Lee Rodwell • Edited by Jim Pollard
Advisory Board: John Chisholm, Sara Richards, Su Wang, Tracy Herd, Clare Greenhalgh • Thanks to all the other women who helped with this publication.
Images: creativecommons.org (Credits p33)
Published: September 2015 • Revision date: September 2018.

ABOUT THIS BOOKLET...

For many years, the Men's Health Forum have published health booklets for men. But customers in the private, public and not-for-profit sectors have all long demanded a title for women to go with our popular Man Manual.

This booklet is the result. Woman was written by a top female health journalist with a female-led editorial and advisory panel. Women of all ages and from all over the UK have been involved in its development. We hope you find it useful.

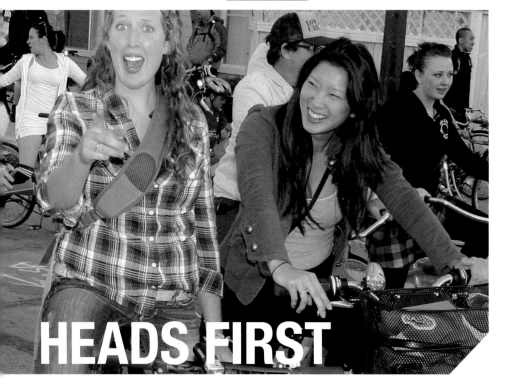

HEADS FIRST

Women can still expect to live longer than men – but the gap is closing.

It's no coincidence that more and more women are now juggling jobs and family responsibilities – and while we care for others, we don't always take as much care of ourselves as we might.

But the good news is that making small changes to the way we live our lives can lead to some big improvements to our health – both now and in the future. This booklet will help you get started.

If you're feeling stressed out, unattractive or unappreciated, what do you do? Head for the biscuit jar, light up a cigarette, pour yourself a glass of wine?

There's a link between the way women feel about themselves and the way they behave – so the first step towards staying healthy is to sort out what's going on in your head.

STRESS-BUSTERS

Being under pressure is part of everyday life – it helps us get things done. But too much stress can affect your health.

If you are caring for others – children or older relatives, for example – it's important to care for yourself too.

> Build some 'me time' into your week to do something you enjoy.

> Learn some deep breathing relaxation techniques or try yoga or tai chi classes.

> Instead of smoking or drinking – which can actually increase anxiety and tension – wind down by reading a magazine or having a soak in the bath.

> Keep up with your friends – phone or message if you can't meet up.

> Switch off the TV, laptop and tablet, get off the sofa and take some exercise – see page 12.

> Eat better – see page 6.

> Set yourself some challenges – learn something new, join a choir, take up painting, become a volunteer.

> Learn how to stand up for yourself and say how you feel – even if that means saying no!

> Identify your stress triggers then find ways to handle pressure better. Could you manage your time better? Would it help to prioritise tasks? Do you need to ask for help?

> Fresh air helps me unwind. I walk the dog or garden.

KNOW YOUR HISTORY

You can get a good idea of the hand you've been dealt by knowing your history.

Many health problems run in families: heart disease, cancer, strokes, depression, mental health challenges.

Find out if your parents, grandparents, aunts and uncles have had any of these illnesses, especially if they died young.

Make sure your GP knows your family health history.

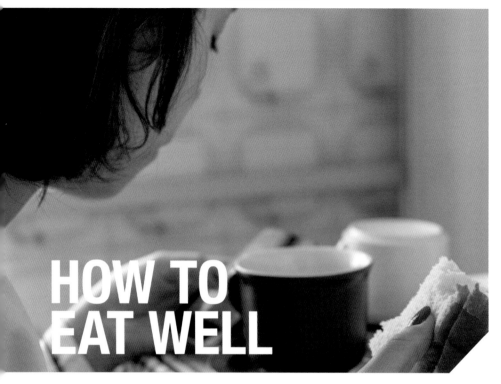

HOW TO EAT WELL

Do you think eating healthily means giving up chocolate forever? Think again.

We need to eat a range of foods to stay healthy – but that doesn't mean we can't have occasional treats. It's just a question of balance.

Eating healthily doesn't have to be complicated. In fact it's quite simple...

JUST EAT MORE...

> fruit and veg

> complex carbs – wholemeal/ wholegrains

> oily fish

AND EAT LESS...

> salt

> saturated fat

> sugar

GET SWAPPING

Some simple swaps can make a big difference.

You could:

> have a spoonful of dried fruit instead of a spoonful of sugar on your breakfast cereal

> swap the frying pan for the grill when cooking meat

> switch from whole milk to skimmed or semi-skimmed.

DON'T BE FOOLED

Be careful about food claims. Do they really mean what you think they do? Learn to read labels and check the fat, salt and sugar content in food when you're shopping and cooking.

Traffic light colours indicate whether a product is high (red), medium (orange) or low (green) in fat, saturates, sugars and salt. Use these to make healthier choices – the more green, the healthier the food is likely to be.

You'll find hidden sugar in some surprising places such as ready meals, soups and ketchup. Salt is also hidden in processed foods, such as bread and breakfast cereals.

'Low fat' doesn't always mean low in calories and foods claiming to be 80% fat-free still have a 20% fat content. Besides, whatever is taken out from food is usually replaced with something else. So low fat foods may be high in sugar and low sugar foods high in fat!

STILL NOT CONVINCED?

> I eat my eggs poached instead of fried.

Here's why what you eat matters:

> Eating healthily can help you feel better – you should have more energy and experience fewer mood swings.

> It reduces the risk of a range of developing diabetes, high blood pressure and high cholesterol and helps to reduce the risk of some cancers and heart disease.

> If you eat well now, you'll stay well longer.

Did you know? Nearly one in 10 UK cancer cases could be prevented through a healthy diet.

HOW MUCH WATER?

I use herbs not salt for flavour.

Drink about 1.6 litres of fluid a day – that's about eight 200ml glasses – but you might need more depending on your size, how active you're being and how hot it is.

And it doesn't have to be water. All drinks count including tea and coffee.

That said, plain water is the healthiest choice.

The sugar in fizzy drinks, squashes, smoothies and fruit juice can lead to weight gain and damage your teeth, so save these for occasional treats. Flavoured waters often contain a lot of sugar, too.

And too much caffeine – found in tea, coffee, and some fizzy drinks – can make you feel anxious and depressed and give you a bad night's sleep.

IT'S NOT HARD TO EAT FIVE A DAY

Lots of people still struggle with the advice to eat at least five portions of fruit and vegetables a day – but here are five quick tips.

> slice a banana on your breakfast cereal

> stir a handful of berries into a low-fat yogurt for a quick pudding

> cook vegetable kebabs and corn cobs when you barbecue

> cut up strips of peppers, cucumber and carrots to eat with a salsa dip

> add chopped carrots and mushrooms to a spaghetti Bolognese.

To cut down on caffeine, I drink herbal tea instead of coffee

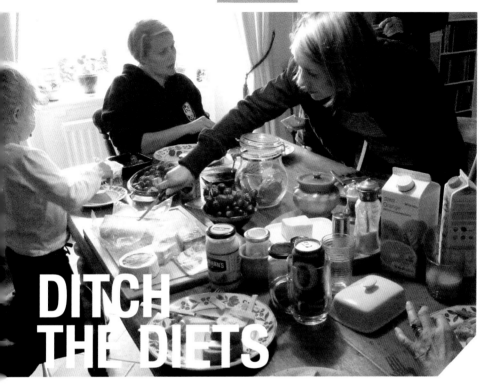

DITCH THE DIETS

How many times have you gone on a diet in order to lose weight before a wedding or to shift the pounds you piled on over Christmas?

And how many times did the weight you lost creep back on again?

The truth is that dieting doesn't work.

Researchers have found that within four or five years at least one-third to two-thirds of dieters have regained more weight than they lost.

And it doesn't seem to matter what kind of diet you follow. One study compared people on a rapid weight loss diet with a group following a gradual weight loss diet. Three years later, seven out of 10 dieters from BOTH groups had regained most of their lost weight.

On top of this, many fad diets – such as the Dukan diet or the Paleo diet – are based on dubious scientific theories or unhealthy ways of eating that can be harmful to health.

Instead of cutting out entire food groups, living on cabbage soup or egg-white omelettes, try making small changes to the way you eat instead.

You could try:

> Eating less.

I keep a bowl of fruit by the sofa - and the biscuits out of sight.

Cook smaller quantities, use smaller plates, take smaller portions, share a pudding. Think twice before having second helpings and don't feel you have to clear your plate.

> Eating more slowly.

Chew your food more. Savour it. Put down your knife and fork between mouthfuls.

> Eating mindfully.

This means focusing on your food. So try not to eat on the go, at your desk, while watching TV or checking your email. Eat at a table if possible and learn to recognise when you're full.

FIVE TOP TIPS

> Stick to a meal routine. Eat at roughly the same time each day (that includes your snacks, if you're a snacker). And don't skip meals – that can lead to overeating later.

> Plan ahead. If you always have an apple or a small pack of dried fruit handy you'll be less likely to buy a packet of crisps or a muffin as a snack.

> Don't eat up leftovers – especially other people's! Put them in the fridge or use left-over vegetables to make a soup.

> Recognise what triggers your snacking. Are you eating to cheer yourself up, or because you're bored?

> Think about other ways you could meet your emotional needs but don't ban treats altogether – you'll just feel deprived and want them even more.

HEALTHY WEIGHT

Doctors use something called the BMI (body mass index) to decide whether someone is a healthy weight or not. But there's an easier way.

Just take a tape measure and measure your waist.

It should be less than half your height.

Even easier, if you want just one figure: 31.5 inches.

As a woman, you have a higher risk of health problems if your waist size is more than 31.5 inches or 80cm (and this risk is even higher if it's more than 34.5 inches or 88cm).

DON'T DETOX

Detox diets usually involve drinking lots of water and cutting out foods such as wheat or dairy products, or fasting for short periods, in order to clear out 'toxins'.

Dieticians say the idea of detox is nonsense because your body filters out, breaks down and gets rid of waste products all the time. That's what your skin, your gut, your liver and your kidneys do.

Of course you need to drink enough water to stay hydrated – but drinking too much water can be dangerous. And eating a balanced diet is better for your health than following a fad.

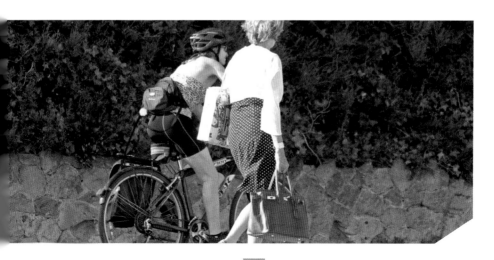

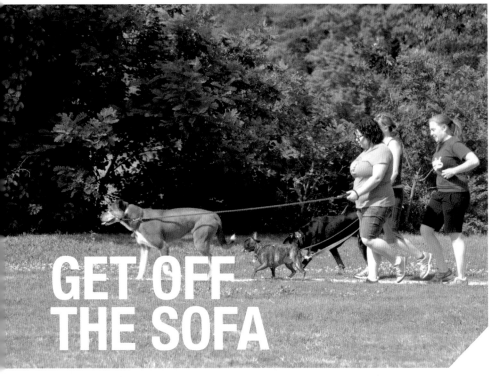

GET OFF THE SOFA

In the UK we spend 60 per cent of our waking hours sitting down.

Are you sitting comfortably? Then stand up and get moving! When it comes to staying healthy, being active is even more important than watching your weight.

You don't have to run marathons or spend hours in the gym. Even a modest amount of exercise – such as a brisk 20 minute walk every day will make a difference, whatever your age.

Being physically active can help you to be healthier – and happier.

As well as reducing the risk of heart disease, type 2 diabetes, stroke, and some cancers, taking regular exercise can also:

> boost your self-esteem

> lift your mood

> give you more energy

> help you sleep better.

Exercise can be beneficial to everyone, but if you have an underlying health condition – such as heart disease or back problems – or if you're pregnant or recovering from an illness, check with your GP before starting anything new.

HOW MUCH EXERCISE?

Try to take some exercise every day.

Aim for at least 150 minutes of moderate-intensity aerobic activity every week. Every little helps – you don't have to do it all in one go.

Moderate-intensity activity – such as walking briskly or cycling on the flat – raises your heart rate and makes you breathe faster and feel warmer. (You're working hard enough if you can still talk, but can't sing the words to a song.)

Vigorous-intensity activity – such as playing singles tennis or running – is even better for your long-term health. (At this level, you won't be able to say more than a few words without pausing for a breath.)

You could do a mix of moderate and vigorous activity: 1 minute of vigorous-intensity activity is about the same as 2 minutes of moderate-intensity activity.

Also, aim to do some muscle-strengthening activities on at least two days a week. You could take up yoga, lift weights in the gym, do push-ups and sit–ups at home – or dig over the garden.

But anything is better than nothing.

WHAT'S STOPPING YOU?

'I'm too tired'

It's a nice paradox that if you get physical instead of flopping on the sofa after a busy day, you will boost your energy levels and feel less tired.

'It's boring'

You don't have to go running or take gym classes. Find something you enjoy – you'll be more likely to keep it up. What about salsa? Or bellydancing?

'I haven't got time'

Are you sure? How much time do you spend on social media or watching TV? Could you get up earlier? See our Five Ways to Get Moving on page 14.

FIVE WAYS TO GET MOVING

1. Slot exercise into your daily routine

> walk the children to school instead of taking the car

> get off your bus/train/tram to work a stop or two early

> use the stairs instead of the lift/escalator at the shopping centre or car park

> mow the lawn or clean the windows

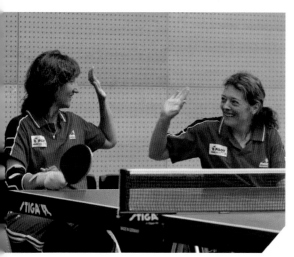

2. Phone a friend

> invite someone to take a class with you

> sign up for a charity walk or run

3. Have fun with your children

> take a Frisbee or a football to the park

> play skipping games

> go on cycle rides

4. Stand up more at home

> hide the TV remote and get up to change channels.

> take out the rubbish in the ad breaks, or get up to tidy the kitchen

5. Stand up more at work

> talk to work colleagues face to face instead of emailing

> stand when making or taking a phone call

DID YOU KNOW? Being physically active can reduce the risk of developing breast, bowel or womb cancer.

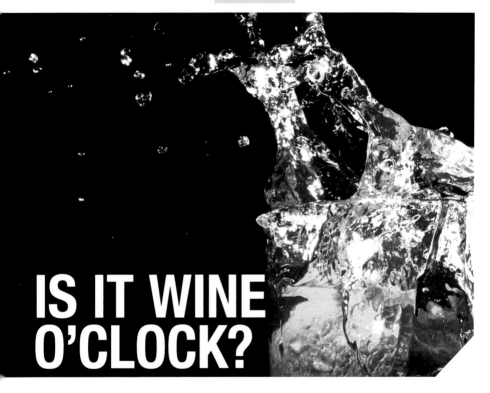

IS IT WINE O'CLOCK?

Some of us like to wind down in the evening with a glass of wine. But before you take your first sip, pause.

Do you know what one unit of alcohol looks like? Probably less than you think.

A glass of wine, for example, is least 2 units – possibly more than 3 depending on the strength of the wine and the size of the glass. Pubs and bars increasingly serve wine in larger glasses – some even contain as much as a third of a bottle!

A pint of beer, lager or cider is also 2-3 units depending on strength.

That's the maximum women are advised to drink in one day.

If you have two or three drinks you could easily consume more than 6 units – almost three times the daily alcohol limit guidelines – without even realising it. And that's classed as binge drinking.

I bought smaller wine glasses to use at home!

There's also a danger in trying to match men drink for drink. The guidelines for women are lower than those for men because women's bodies don't process alcohol as well.

Women have a higher ratio of fat to water than men, so they are less able to dilute alcohol in the body. Women also tend to have lower levels than men of the chemical that metabolises alcohol in the liver.

And as women get older they become even more sensitive to alcohol's effects.

Alcohol can:

> affect fertility

> put you at greater risk of breast cancer

> affect your appearance

> contribute to weight gain

> disrupt your sleep

> increase some side effects of the menopause

I sleep so much better now I've stopped drinking during the week.

And although it may not be apparent for years, drinking over the lower limit guidelines most days or every day can cause a whole range of health problems including liver disease and several types of cancer.

Sounds scary, doesn't it? But there are plenty of ways you can cut down on your alcohol intake, safeguard your health and still enjoy yourself.

EIGHT WAYS TO CUT BACK

1. Find alternative stress-busters

Instead of having a drink to wind down at the end of the day, have a cup of herbal tea or go and soak in the bath.

2. Take a break

Have alcohol-free days. Build up to having an alcohol-free week or month. Note the benefits – are you sleeping better, do you have more energy?

3. Switch to lower alcohol drinks

Check the label for the ABV (alcoholic strength by volume) or ask the bar staff. The lower the better. A lower alcohol wine, for example, might have an ABV of 5.5% instead of the usual 12-14%.

4. Become a mixologist

Have a mocktail instead of a cocktail. You'll find plenty of recipes online. Try a Virgin Mohito. In a tall glass, crush a handful of fresh mint leaves with a teaspoon of brown sugar. Add crushed ice and top up with low calorie lemonade. Garnish with a sprig of mint and a slice of lime.

5. Dilute your drinks.

Have a white wine spritzer or a shandy made with low calorie lemonade.

6. Sit at a table in the pub or wine bar

People drink more quickly when they are standing.

7. Don't finish the bottle

If you're sharing a bottle with a partner or friend, don't feel you have to drink it all. Screw the top back on or push the cork back in and it should keep for a couple of days. Or try a wine box – they last for weeks.

8. Keep tabs on those units

Download the NHS Drinks Tracker app to your phone so you can see how much you're drinking. It's free from the iTunes App Store or from Google Play.

WHAT'S IN YOUR GLASS?

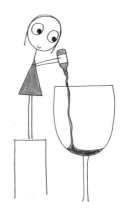

The calories in alcohol have no nutritional value – they're empty calories. Alcoholic drinks are also full of sugar. So spending an evening drinking is like spending an evening eating cakes!

Pint of cider (4.5% ABV) = 1 doughnut (210 calories)

Large glass of wine (250ml, 13% ABV) = 1 Cornetto (228 cals)

Standard glass wine (175ml, 13% ABV) = 1 slice angel layer cake (160 cals)

Glass of champagne (125ml, 12% ABV) = 2 Jaffa cakes (89 cals)

Single gin (25ml, 40% ABV) and slimline tonic = 1 Cadbury Mini roll (115 cals)

A pint of cider contains as many as five teaspoons of sugar – almost as much as the recommended upper daily limit. While two glasses of white wine provide 360 calories – nearly one fifth of a woman's daily calorie allowance.

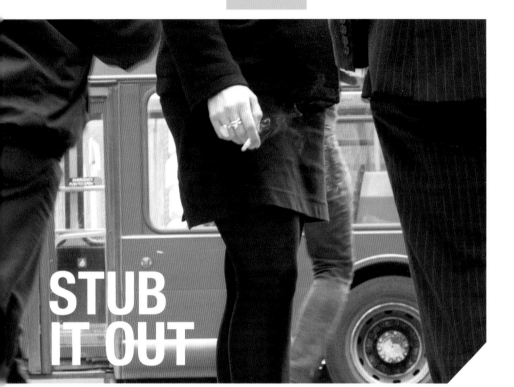

STUB IT OUT

If you smoke, quitting is likely to be the most important step you can take to improve your health. As well as increasing the risk of a heart attack or stroke, smoking can cause at least 14 types of cancer – including ovarian and cervical cancer.

You will start to see some benefits very quickly – and you'll be adding years to your life and greatly improving your prospects of enjoying a healthy, mobile, happier old age. But long before that…

> You'll feel less stressed. Nicotine addiction makes smokers experience a 'withdrawal' between cigarettes. The pleasant feeling when you satisfy that craving is only temporary and is not a real cure for stress.

> Your skin will look less sallow and your face will age less slowly with fewer lines and wrinkles.

> Your teeth won't become stained and your breath won't smell stale.

> Your sex life could improve. You may become aroused more easily and have stronger orgasms.

> Your sense of taste and smell will improve.

> You'll have more puff and energy so you'll be able to run for a bus or keep up with the kids in the park.

> Your fertility levels will improve. Quitting also makes it less likely that you will miscarry and increases your chance of having a healthy baby.

> You'll be less likely to get gum disease.

> Your immune system will work better making it easier for you to fight off colds and flu.

Stopping smoking at the age of 30 increases life expectancy by 10 years. But it's never too late to benefit.

Ring the Smokefree National Helpline (number on page 34) for information and/or referral to the free NHS stop smoking services.

WHAT ARE YOU WEIGHT-ING FOR?

Some smokers gain weight when they quit because nicotine affects appetite and metabolism. But weight gain isn't inevitable if you eat healthily and take some exercise.

Giving up cigarettes means you'll be able to breathe better and you'll probably have more energy, so exercising will be easier and more enjoyable. In any case, putting on weight is less of a health risk than continuing to smoke.

Nicotine is highly addictive but you can double your chance of quitting successfully if you use products such as patches, lozenges, inhalers, and/or gum that contain nicotine. The idea is to wean yourself off nicotine by gradually reducing your intake until you don't need it any more.

WHAT ABOUT E-CIGARETTES?

Electronic cigarettes contain nicotine as well as other chemicals and flavourings but because they don't contain any tobacco, they are seen as much less harmful than smoking. There is evidence that using e-cigarettes – or vaping – can help smokers quit altogether. However, the step between smoking and not smoking is smaller when you vape, so it may be easier to slip back into the habit.

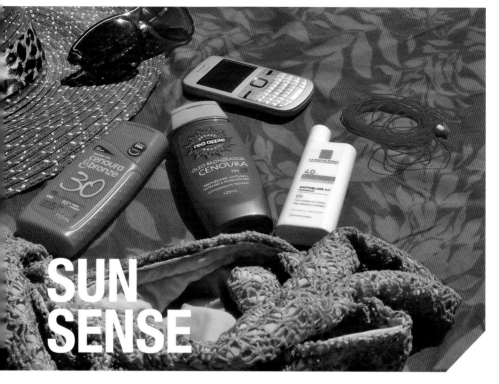

SUN SENSE

Is the sun good or bad for us? It can be both.

Sunlight is our main source of Vitamin D, which is essential for strong bones.

Low levels are linked to conditions like osteoporosis (brittle bones) and there's evidence that Vitamin D may also help to protect us from getting cancer, heart disease, diabetes, multiple sclerosis and other chronic diseases.

BUT exposure to sunlight is also the main cause of skin cancer and it can age your skin prematurely.

So how can you enjoy the sun safely? The two key things to remember are:

> Little and often is best

> Never burn

This is even more important if you have fair skin that burns easily, light-coloured eyes or lots of moles or freckles.

Keep sunscreen handy so you're never caught out by the sun.

When the sun is strong or you're at risk of burning:

> Spend time in the shade

> Cover up with clothing and wear sunglasses and a hat with a peak or brim

> Use a sunscreen

When your shadow is shorter than you are, the sun is more likely to burn you.

YES TO SUNSCREEN

Go for a sunscreen with a protection level of at least SPF 15 and 4 stars. Use it generously and reapply regularly.

Make sure it's not past its expiry date – most have a shelf life of 2-3 years.

Remember that sweating, going in water and drying off with a towel can remove sunscreen – even the ones that claim to last for eight hours or more.

Don't rely on your facial moisturiser even if it has an SPF 15. You won't have applied it thickly enough – and won't be reapplying regularly through the day.

YES TO SHADES

Too much exposure to sunlight – especially reflected from water or snow – can damage your eyes. Play it safe in the sun by wearing a hat that shades your face and sunglasses.

Not all sunglasses are up to the job. Don't just focus on style or price – make sure you choose a pair that has wide or wraparound arms to protect the sides of your eyes and one or more of the following: the CE Mark and British Standard (BS EN 1836:2005); a UV 400 label; or, a statement that the sunglasses offer 100% UV protection.

NO TO SUNBEDS

When you use a sunbed your skin is exposed to harmful UV rays that increase your risk skin cancer and other problems such as cataracts.

If you want to look tanned, the safest way is to use a fake tan. But this won't protect your skin from sunburn so you will still need to use sunscreen when you are in the sun.

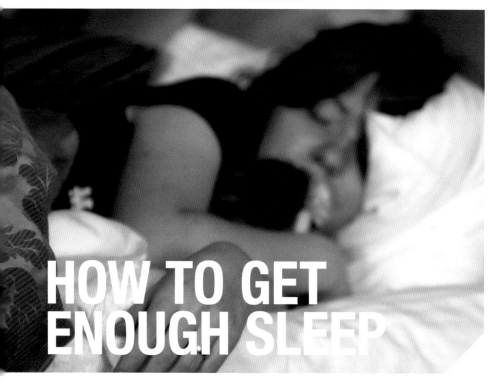

HOW TO GET ENOUGH SLEEP

One in three Britons sometimes has trouble sleeping. And women suffer more than men.

A snoring partner. Wakeful children. Worries about work. The end result? A bad night's sleep.

Most of us have to deal with an occasional broken or restless night that leaves us feeling grumpy and tired the next day. But regularly sleeping badly could have serious consequences for your health.

Of course, the reverse is also true. Sleeping well can help you live a long and healthy life.

DID YOU KNOW? Blue light from smart phones, tablets and e-readers can slow or prevent the production of the sleep hormone melatonin.

HOW MUCH SLEEP?

Everyone is different. It mainly depends on your age, but also your lifestyle.

Most adults need around eight hours sleep each night. Some people can get by with much less. If you are awake and alert throughout the day, you're probably getting enough. If you wake up feeling tired and grumpy, and/or feel sleepy during the day, you're probably not.

If you're having trouble sleeping, you've probably developed some bad bedroom habits.

TEN SIMPLE SLEEP TACTICS

1. Set your alarm clock

Get in the habit of going to bed and getting up at roughly the same time every day. Don't sleep in after a bad night – it will make it harder to get to sleep the following night.

2. Cut down on caffeine

Caffeine – found in tea, coffee and some fizzy drinks – is a stimulant that stays in your body for hours and can keep you awake. So avoid anything with caffeine in for six hours before bedtime.

3. Go for a walk

Moderate, regular exercise such as swimming or walking, can help relieve tension and make it easier to sleep. The best time to exercise is late afternoon or early evening. Later than this may disturb your sleep. This doesn't mean you can't have sex, though!

4. Avoid alcohol in the evening

It may help you fall asleep, but you will almost certainly wake in the night because alcohol affects the quality of sleep and acts as a diuretic (so you'll need to get up to go to the loo).

5. Eat earlier – but don't go to bed hungry

Have your evening meal earlier rather than later but don't go to bed hungry – if necessary, have a light snack.

6. Get the temperature right

Turn down the heating thermostat or open your bedroom window. If it's too hot – or too cold – you won't sleep well. Researchers say a temperature between 60F and 67F (16C to 19C) is optimal for sleeping.

7. Switch off early

Don't check emails, watch TV or message friends right up until bedtime. If you want to read in bed, pick up a paperback not an e-reader or tablet.

8. Block out the world

Make your bedroom as quiet and dark as possible. Try using an eye mask or ear plugs.

9. Unburden yourself

Deal with worries or a heavy workload by making a 'to do' list and tell yourself you'll deal with things tomorrow.

10. Wind down to bedtime

Have a warm (not hot) bath, listen to quiet music or do some relaxation exercises.

If none of this helps, and lack of sleep is affecting your daily life, see your GP

Your doctor can check that your sleeplessness is not due to a physical illness, any medicines you're taking, or emotional problems. He or she may refer you for CBT – cognitive behaviour therapy – rather than prescribing sleeping tablets as these don't work for long and are addictive.

CBT is a talking treatment that helps you examine the thoughts that affect your feelings and behaviour and teaches skills to deal with problems.

OVER THE COUNTER SLEEP REMEDIES

Always check with your GP or a pharmacist before using sleeping remedies. They often contain an antihistamine that will make you sleepy but may leave you still feeling drowsy the next day.

Herbal medicines usually contain Valerian. Research isn't clear on the benefits and there may be side effects such as headaches.

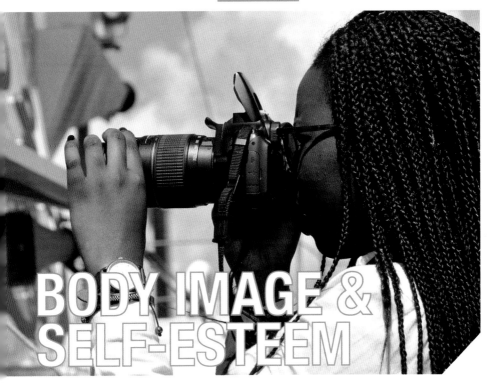

BODY IMAGE & SELF-ESTEEM

Eight out of 10 women agree that every woman has something about her that is beautiful – but do not see their own beauty.

Be as nice to yourself as you are to those you love.

When you look in the mirror do you like what you see? Or do you simply notice things you wish you could change? Having a positive body image will boost your self-esteem and help you to be healthier and happier. Here's how:

> Focus on what you like about your body and pay yourself a compliment. Say: "My legs look great in these jeans." Or: "I have really glossy hair."

> Instead of only thinking about the way your body looks, think about what it can do. Tell yourself: "These strong arms do front crawl." Or: "These legs can take me for long walks."

> Find ways to silence your inner critic, the voice in your head that tells you you're flabby, or silly, or not good enough. Imagine the voice is a parrot in a

cage. Every time you hear a squawk, imagine yourself throwing a cloth over the cage to send the parrot to sleep.

> Think positive thoughts and list some of your strengths – like making great lasagne or being a good listener. Keep the list where you can see it – on your fridge, at your desk – and add to it regularly.

WHEN HOME ISN'T A SAFE PLACE

More than 1 in 4 women have experienced some kind of domestic abuse

It's not just about being punched or kicked: domestic abuse can be physical, psychological, sexual or financial.

It covers threats, shoves and pushes, hair-pulling, constant criticism, stopping you from seeing family or friends – it's any kind of controlling behaviour by a family member that frightens you or undermines your self esteem.

If this is happening to you, remember you are not alone and it is not your fault.

Whether you would simply like someone to talk to, or specific information about how to stay safe, check the list on page 34 to find organisations that offer advice and support.

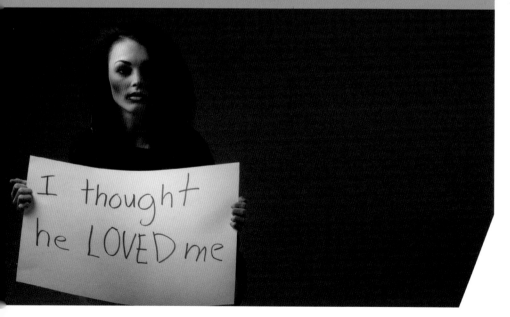

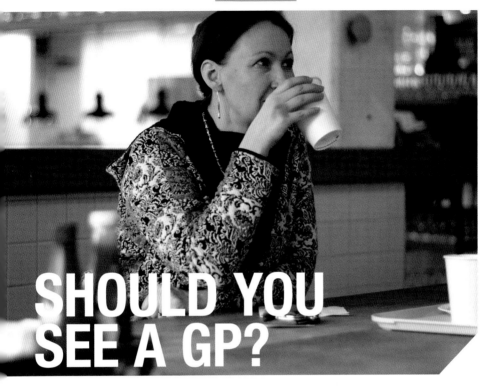

SHOULD YOU SEE A GP?

URINARY TRACT INFECTIONS

One in two women will have a urinary tract infection at least once during their life.

Lessen the risk of getting a UTI by:

> emptying your bladder after sex

> wiping from front to back after going to the toilet

> avoiding constipation.

Urinary tract infections usually get better on their own within four or five days. But you should see your GP the first time you have these symptoms or if you have a UTI more than three times in one year.

You should also see a GP if you develop a high temperature, your symptoms suddenly get worse, you are pregnant or have diabetes.

Don't be afraid to ask silly questions - it's only silly not to ask.

STRESS INCONTINENCE

One in three women in the UK leak a little when they laugh or sneeze. Lessen the risk of stress incontinence by:

> doing pelvic floor exercises regularly, especially during pregnancy

> staying a healthy weight

> not smoking

If you are a lady who leaks, don't suffer in embarrassed silence. Talk to your GP who will discuss treatment options with you.

HOW TO DO PELVIC FLOOR EXERCISES

Make yourself comfortable, either standing or sitting tall. Now squeeze and lift the muscles you would use if you were trying to stop yourself weeing and passing wind at the same time.

You should feel your vagina and back passage drawing up inside and your lower abdominal muscles should also be working.

Try not to hold your breath or tighten your stomach, buttock or thigh muscles.

When you get used to doing this, hold each squeeze for a few seconds, then release and rest.

Every week, you can add more squeezes and hold each for as long as you can (up to 10 seconds), then release and rest for a few seconds.

Don't give up – it may take a few months before you notice the results.

THRUSH

Most women experience occasional bouts of thrush – itching, soreness and swelling of the vagina caused by a yeast infection – particularly during pregnancy or after a course of antibiotics.

To lessen the risk of getting thrush:

> wash your vaginal area with water and avoid perfumed soaps, shower gels, vaginal deodorants, or douches

> avoid latex condoms, spermicidal creams or lubricants if they irritate your genital area

> wearing cotton underwear, not synthetics

> avoiding tights, leggings and skinny jeans

See a GP the first time you get thrush for a swab to confirm the diagnosis. After that, if you recognize the symptoms, you can just go to a pharmacy and buy anti-thrush medication over the counter.

If the thrush doesn't clear up, or if you have frequent bouts (at least one every few months), see your GP again.

Vaginal thrush isn't an STI, but it can sometimes be passed on to men during sex. Men can have thrush without noticing it, so if you are in a relationship and keep getting attacks, you could be treating your thrush and then your partner could be giving it straight back to you.

Thrush can also be triggered by sex, especially if your vagina is too dry.

PERIOD PROBLEMS

If your periods change, it doesn't necessarily mean there's a serious problem – but it should be investigated.

So if you notice you're bleeding between periods or after sex, or if your periods become heavier or longer, see your doctor.

If your periods have stopped (and you're not pregnant), or if they're heavy, irregular or very painful, talk to your GP about treatments that could help.

PREMENSTRUAL SYNDROME (PMS)

Nearly all women have some premenstrual symptoms from bloating to mood swings. But 5-10% get PMS which is severe enough to prevent them from getting on with their daily lives. Improve your symptoms by:

> taking more exercise

> eating a healthy balanced diet

> avoiding caffeine and alcohol

> drinking plenty of water

> finding ways to reduce stress

If PMS disrupts your life, discuss lifestyle changes and treatments with your GP.

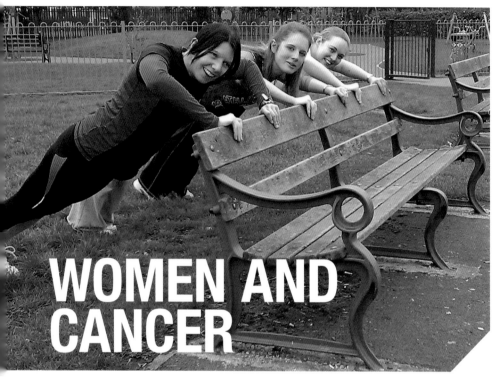

WOMEN AND CANCER

No one likes to think about cancer, but there's no getting away from it – half of us in the UK will develop cancer at some point in our lives.

It's not all bad news. Cancer may be more common – but more people are surviving cancer than ever before. Take breast cancer for example: survival rates have doubled in the UK in the last 40 years.

Cancer Research UK say that more than four out of 10 cases of cancer can be prevented by making the kind of lifestyle changes this booklet suggests. But women also need to be vigilant – and not only for signs of the cancers that we associate with being female.

Lung cancer is still the biggest ladykiller, followed by breast cancer. Third comes bowel cancer, responsible for one in 10 of all female cancer deaths.

That sounds scary. But the sooner cancer is diagnosed, the easier it is to treat – and the more likely treatment will be successful.

So accept invitations for 'smear' tests and mammograms to screen for cervical and breast cancer even if you think everything is fine (and don't panic if you are recalled – in many cases, there will be nothing to worry about.)

But also get to know your body and what's normal for you. Keep an eye out for any unusual, persistent changes and if you notice a change, talk it over with your practice nurse or doctor.

THE PILL AND CANCER

Taking the pill increases the risk of breast and cervical cancer – but the combined contraceptive pill lowers the risk of ovarian and womb cancer, and may also lower the risk of bowel cancer.

Experts agree that any increase in risk is likely to be small and starts to drop as soon as you come off the pill. After 10 years the risk is the same as if you had never taken it.

BREAST CANCER: SEVEN SIGNS TO WATCH FOR

Breast cancer is easily the most common cancer in women – but the good news is that more women are surviving breast cancer than ever before.

The key is to catch it early. Be breast aware. Watch out for:

1. A lump or thickening in an area of the breast

2. A change in the size or shape of your breast

3. Dimpling of the skin like orange peel

4. A change in the shape of a nipple

5. Discharge from one or both nipples

6. Redness or a rash on the skin and/or around the nipple

7. A swelling or lump in your armpit

These signs don't necessarily mean cancer – most lumps are harmless. But if you notice any change from what is normal for you, see your GP as soon as possible.

DID YOU KNOW? Having 1 drink a day could increase the risk of breast cancer by 5%. And the risk increases the more a woman drinks.

ANTIPERSPIRANTS AND BREAST CANCER

Parabens are chemicals used in deodorants and antiperspirants, as well as many other cosmetic products.

Parabens have been found in breast tissue removed following breast cancer but researchers haven't found any convincing evidence that parabens cause breast cancer.

Sometimes women are advised not to use deodorants containing aluminium salts before going for breast screening.

This isn't because the salts are dangerous, but because they can affect the results of screening tests and make breast cancers harder to detect.

CERVICAL CANCER

Women of all ages can develop cancer in the cervix – the neck of the womb – but it's the most common cancer in women under 35. Most cases are linked to the human papillomavirus (HPV) which can be spread during sexual activity, so using a condom can reduce your risk of infection.

There are now vaccines to prevent HPV infection but they don't protect against all types of the virus and it will be some time before the vaccination programme will reduce the number of cervical cancer cases.

That's why it is important to go for cervical screening – commonly known as having a 'smear' test. (You need to be registered with a GP to be invited for screening.)

If you are too young – or too old – to be called for screening, watch out for:

> any unusual bleeding from the vagina, particularly after sex or after the menopause

> persistent vaginal discharge that is blood-stained or smells unpleasant

These can be early signs of cervical cancer.

Even if you've had a normal screening result or been vaccinated against HPV, it's important to let your doctor know if you develop any of these signs so they can be checked out straight away.

DID YOU KNOW? The best time to have a 'smear' test is in the middle of your menstrual cycle because the health professional is likely to get the best possible sample of cells at this time.

WOMB CANCER

Womb cancer is almost always curable if caught at an early stage.

The early symptoms are:

> vaginal bleeding after the menopause

> bleeding that is unusually heavy or happens between periods

> vaginal discharge, from pink and watery to dark and foul smelling

These can also be symptoms of much more common conditions than womb cancer but if you have any of them, it's important to see your doctor to find out.

Don't die of embarrassment. Doctors have seen it all before.

OVARIAN CANCER

When ovarian cancer is diagnosed at an early stage, the outcome is usually good. If you know the key signs to look out for, you can seek advice as soon as possible.

These are:

> persistent pelvic and abdominal pain

> increased abdominal size/persistent bloating

> difficulty eating and feeling full quickly

If you regularly have any of these symptoms – and they are not normal for you – see your GP, particularly if you are over 50 or have a strong family history of breast or ovarian cancer.

PHOTO CREDITS: Thanks to Aidan-Sally, Bruno Padhila, Cave Coillier, dualdflipflop, FaceMePLS, Gaël Marziou, Pam Loves Pie, Quinn Dombrowski, Richard Masoner, Shélin Graziela, starsandspirals, Tony Alter, Alexander Baxevanis and Vikram Vetrival who were all kind enough to make their images available through the Creative Commons. (If this is not the case, please contact us.) Full credits, links and licences at: menshealthforum.org.uk/MMreferences

WHO CAN HELP?

NHS CHOICES

Online 'front door' to NHS
www.nhs.uk
www.nhs.uk/change4life
apps.nhs.uk
Call 111 (24 hour) for non-emergency medical advice.
http://tinyurl.com/oohNHS for more on NHS out of hours.

EATING AND DRINKING

British Dietetic Association
www.bda.uk.com
British Nutrition Foundation
www.nutrition.org.uk
Drinkaware
drinkaware.co.uk

NHS Choices
www.nhs.uk/livewell www.
The NHS has a Drinks Tracker app. Or text Units to 64746 to access the NHS alcohol units calculator on any smartphone

Alcoholic Anonymous
0845 769 7555
www.alcoholics-anonymous.co.uk

CANCER

Breast Cancer Care
www.breastcancercare.org.uk
Helpline 0808 800 6000
Cancer Research UK
www.cancerresearchuk.org
The Eve Appeal
www.eveappeal.org.uk
Macmillan Cancer
Free helpline   0808 808 00 00
www.macmillan.org.uk

DOMESTIC VIOLENCE

Refuge
www.refuge.org.uk
Women's Aid
www.womensaid.org.uk
National Domestic Violence Helpline
0808 2000 247

CONTRACEPTION AND SEXUAL HEALTH

fpa
www.fpa.org.uk

MENTAL WELLBEING

Mental Health Foundation
www.mentalhealth.org.uk
Mind
www.mind.org.uk

SMOKING

Smokefree
www.smokefree.nhs.co.uk

Ring the Smokefree National Helpline on 0300 123 1044 for information and/or referral to the free NHS stop smoking services in England. The number for Scotland is 0800 848484, and for Wales 0800 085 2219.

BLADDER AND BOWEL

Bladder and Bowel Foundation
bladderandbowelfoundation.org
Beating Bowel Cancer
www.beatingbowelcancer.org
The IBS Network (irritable bowel syndrome)
www.theibsnetwork.org
The Cystitis and Overactive Bladder Foundation
www.cobfoundation.org

FEELING DESPERATE?

Samaritans   08457 90 90 90
Emotional support 24/7
www.samaritans.org

The authors and the publisher have taken care to make sure that the advice given in this edition is correct at the time of publication. We advise you to read and understand the instructions and information included with all medicines and to carefully consider whether a treatment is worth taking. The authors and the publisher have no legal responsibility for the results of treatments, misuse or overuse of the remedies in this book or their level of success in individual cases.

The author and the publisher do not intend this book to be used instead of advice from a medical practitioner, which you should always get for any symptom or illness.